Low Sugar Smoothies

50 Sugar Free Smoothies

© 2015 by Peggy Annear
Published by Kangaroo Flat Books

ISBN – 13: 978-1507890097

ISBN -10: 1507890095

If you would like a linked, Kindle or PC full Color Copy of this book please visit the author's page.

www.amazon.com/author/peggy-annear

Table of Contents

The Smoothie Advantage! 7

Why Low Sugar Smoothies? 9

Best Low Sugar Ingredients for Smoothies 11

Counting Carbs in Fruit & Vegetables................................. 13

Beware of Low Fat Foods... 15

Superfood Booster List 17

About the Recipes 19

Green Smoothie Blends 23

Basic Green Smoothie Blend 25

Green Blackberry Smoothie 26

Mango & Kale Green Smoothie................................. 27

Berry Delight... 28

Healing Smoothie.. 29

Slimming Smoothie.. 30

Kale Mojito 31

Pink Cabbage Glow.. 32

Green Vegetable Bomb 33

Green Light Smoothie 34

V8 Juice... 35

Refreshing Mango Melon Smoothie 36

Cinnaberry Green Smoothie..................................... 37

Peanut Butter and Jelly Smoothie 38

Vitamin C Blast 39

Kiwi Spinach Smoothie 40

Vanilla Parsley Smoothie 41

Green Pumpkin Smoothie 42

Coconut Pear Smoothie 43

Emerald Green Smoothie 44

David's Super Smoothie 45

Dairy Smoothie Blends 47

Low GI Oat Drink 49

Milky Blackberry Green Smoothie 50

Iced Coffee Smoothie 51

Peaches & Cream 52

Eggnog Smoothie 53

Smoothie Tropicana 54

Two Color Smoothie 55

Almond Cacao Crunch 56

Berry Cocoa Smoothie 57

Sunset Cabbage Blend 58

Strawberry Cream Protein Smoothie 59

Green Pumpkin Smoothie 60

Fruit, Vegetable & Protein Smoothie Blends 61

Carrot and Orange Smoothie 63

Protein Shake 64

Sparkling Peach Wine 65

Carrot Cake Frappe 66

Blueberry Smoothie 67

Green Avocado Blaster 68

Protein Hot Chocolate 69

Bloody Mary Smoothie 70

Spirulina Vanilla Protein Smoothie.. 71

Strawberry Thick Shake 72

Green Tea Smoothie... 73

Super Smoothie 74

Easy Tomato Squash 75

High Protein Smoothie... 76

Smooth Ruby.. 77

Mint Protein Thick Shake 78

Homemade Coconut Milk Recipe 79

Helpful Resources 80

Notes.. 82

The Smoothie Advantage!

Healthy smoothies benefit our bodies and our lives in numerous ways. Here are a few common advantages.

- Rich in nutrients, vitamins and oils
- Contains healthy dietary fat required for burning energy and healthy biological functions
- Low sugar, high alkaline greens help detox and reduce inflammation
- Assists with keeping the body hydrated
- Assists in weight loss and even healthy meal replacement
- Preparation, consumption and digestion are simple
- High fibre - constipation can be a thing of the past!
- Healthy all-in-one quick low sugar meal when you are busy!

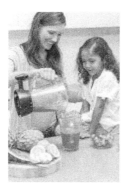

Start the morning with a delicious fresh breakfast smoothie that's not only loaded with vitamins, antioxidants, healthy fats and protein but tastes amazing! Use fresh fruits and vegetables that are in season. These will not only save you money, but taste a lot better too.

Remember, if the ingredients are wilting or not ripe, the taste will be compromised. If you have a powerful blender, you can choose to add a few harder ingredients such as dried fruits, dark 70% Cacao+ chocolate, nuts and seeds.

Purchase organic fruits, or locally grown if possible. Wash or peel the fruits and vegetables first.

Why Low Sugar Smoothies?

Some people begin to make low sugar smoothies to lose weight, while others watch their Diabetes or just want to lead a healthier lifestyle and have more energy. If you get the smoothie balance right, you will have an abundance of energy due to drinking a beverage packed with nutrition. Don't waste money buying sports or protein drinks, making your own natural, fresh smoothies not only tastes better but is a whole lot cheaper too. It is even possible to freeze smoothies and take them with us while out and on the go.

Reducing sugar from your diet is the quickest way to lose fat and boost your energy levels. You can eat as many green vegetables as you desire, so making smoothies is a good way to incorporate more greens into your diet.

Making smoothies is a hit at our house because they are fast to make, flexible with the ingredients used, and they are nutritious. They can also save you money if you buy fruits or vegetables on special at the supermarket, or if you have an abundance from your own garden. Of course when people are on their way to work or kids are off to school, smoothies are perfect for that quick to prepare meal or snack.

When making low sugar smoothies, a good rule of thumb is to be aware of and limit the amount of ALL sweeteners used including fruits. That being said, there is no point making all vegetable or green smoothies that taste so horrible you decide to abandon smoothie making entirely. This is especially true of beginners or if you are introducing green smoothies or low sugar smoothies to your children. Common sense must prevail. Once you learn the basic concept of which low sugar food blends are best for you dietary needs the smoothie combinations will come to you more easily. Alter the sweetness taste to suit yourself and aim to reduce it slightly over time for better health. Of course adding processed sugar is OUT altogether as it contains no nutritional benefit whatsoever and has a negative impact on our health in many ways. Learn how to read food labels correctly and more about the "No Sugar Diet" in my book. There is a 7 Day Detox Plan and a list of 30 Smoothie Detox Super Foods included to get you started. This book also looks at the pitfalls of trying to incorporate artificial sweeteners as a long term solution.

Although vegetables and fruits are natural, be cautious of using too many high sugary fruits, honey and dates. Yes, we need to have some sweetening to make our smoothies palatable, it's all about balance. If I make a smoothie and it seems too sweet, I will cut down on the fruits. For example, if you want to add dates as your sweetener to a smoothie, only add a few to a vegetable smoothie to keep the low sugar balance. Some people find smoothies useful for fasting or as a meal replacement.

These easy to make, nourishing smoothies are great for adults and kids of all ages. You can play around with many of the ingredients and come up with your own favorites. You can leave things out or add some new ones if you prefer a particular taste. That's what I love about them, they are so changeable but still so tasty and nutritious.

Best Low Sugar Ingredients for Smoothies

Raspberries, strawberries, blackberries, limes, under ripe bananas, tomato and lemons are about the lowest in natural sugars while also being good for smoothie making. Spinach and kale are excellent greens in low sugar smoothies and blend up easily. All salad greens are excellent, as are celery and capsicum. Carrots are also good with some sweetness. While you probably cannot always use these ingredients, you may try incorporating them into your diet regularly.

Try to incorporate foods from the following super-food list where possible for general health and warding off sickness.

Counting Carbs in Fruit & Vegetables

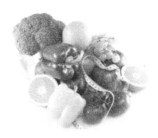

Foods that have less than 5g sugar per 100g are considered low sugar foods. Foods that have more than 15g sugar per 100g are high sugar foods. Of course varieties and brands vary in sugar/carbohydrate content. If you want to control how much sugar is added via liquids such as milks and juices, it is important to educate yourself by reading the Nutritional Facts on food labels. This is explained more thoroughly in my No Sugar Diet book. While only some foods are suitable for smoothies, here is a general guide to get you started. It gets down to **balance and proportion to make your smoothie palatable**.

Do your own Google research on a computer; type in" how much sugar" (or carbs) are in (vegetables - select from the drop down box)

Vegetables Lowest in Sugars and Suitable for Smoothies

- Spinach
- Kale
- Zucchini
- Salad greens
- Broccoli
- Cauliflower

Fruits Lowest in Sugars and Suitable for Smoothies:

- Lemons
- Limes
- Strawberries
- Blackberries
- Watermelon

- Kiwifruit
- Grapefruit (for the brave)
- Oranges
- Peaches
- Under ripe bananas
- Avocado
- Tomatoes

Beware of Low Fat Foods

Read labels carefully when shopping in the supermarket because low fat products can be loaded with sugars to put flavor back into a bland tasting product. An example of this is commonly found in low fat yoghurts, low fat milks, low fat creams, ice cream and cookies. Watch for unsweetened products and read labels if using store bought. While some of the recipes call for almond or coconut milk, read labels carefully and be sure they are not laced with sugar! Certain low fat milks and almond milk varieties can be extremely sweet, so beware!

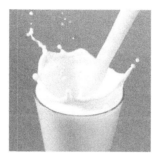

Use plain water, natural unsweetened milks, creams and coconut water to mix your smoothies. If weight loss is your goal, aim for low fat, low sugar combinations. A tip: The Google Search Method I use is "how much sugar is in..." to discover sugar levels in different foods. Likewise, this can be done for "how much fat is in..."

Carbohydrates are the body's main source of energy and during digestion, sugar which is simple carbohydrates, and starches which are complex carbohydrates, break down into blood sugar also known as glucose. Consuming too much food that is high in carbohydrates can quickly spike blood sugar levels which may cause problems over time. Monitoring and maintaining carbohydrate intake is key to blood sugar control.

Superfood Booster List

Create your own low sugar super smoothie recipes. Use this basic natural super-food list as a guide. A balance of sweet and savory will make it tasty! Some are for the brave, so experiment; add a little at a time.

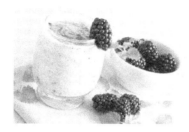

- Cabbage is good for the stomach and treating peptic ulcers. Chinese cabbage has a mild flavor.
- Leafy green vegetable smoothies are packed with antioxidants and vital nutrients. They also help lower the acidity levels and inflammation in our body.
- Beets are good for cleansing the liver, gall bladder and bowel.
- Berries are not only relatively low sugar fruits but they are also high in phytochemicals which are naturally occurring nutrients that help protect cells from damage.
- Natural sweeteners can be used such as soaked dates, raisins, and prunes. Date sugar, maple syrup, carob powder and raw honey are also good.
- Apple and pineapple juice are good to help cover up an unpleasant taste.
- Cayenne pepper is good for circulation.
- Alfalfa is good for bowel health.
- Anise (herb) will help reduce gas in the stomach.
- Citrus fruits, and any fruit/veg high in ascorbic acid help boost the immune system and fight cancer.
- Carrots contain beta-carotene, which help fight infection and cancer.
- Coriander (cilantro) is good for the heart and the digestive system.
- Dandelion is a mild diuretic.

- Echinacea is a good detoxifying agent for cleaning the lymphatic system.
- Figs and prunes are a natural laxative
- Grapes are a good blood purifier.
- Kale is high in calcium and good for our teeth and bones.
- Lemons, oranges and grapefruit help eliminate catarrh, and boost immune system.
- Mangoes are good for the intestines.
- Milk (cows) is a complete protein.
- Lettuce can slow digestion, but is good for insomnia.
- Parsley is a tonic for the kidneys and blood vessels.
- Mint is good to help cover a "yucky" taste and also good for digestion.
- Pineapple is a good source of manganese and vitamin C, great for the blood and digestion.
- Pomegranate is good for urinary problems and is a detox blood cleanser.
- Papaya is good for intestinal disorders.
- Radish is good for catarrh.
- Sage is a good "wake up" herb and also good for the sinuses.
- Spinach is great raw in drinks, but don't overdo it because it contains oxalic acid.
- Spirulina is an algae that is rich in protein and can help boost your immune system and regulate cholesterol.
- Thyme helps alleviate headaches, asthma and cold symptoms.
- Watermelon is good for the kidneys and is a blood cooler, great for summer.
- Watercress helps eliminate fluids from the body because it is high in potassium.
- Wheatgrass is high in Indole which helps prevent cancer. It is high in many beneficial.

- Oatmeal only contains 0.3g sugar per 100g with 17g per 100g of protein! Also great for thickening smoothies.
- Nuts are FULL of the good oils!
- Natural protein boosters for weight gain and vitality include egg yolk, nut butters, ground nuts and seeds, milks, soy powder, good quality unsweetened protein powders and cottage cheese.

About the Recipes

Basic Smoothie Making Tips

- Buy fresh fruits and vegetables that are in season for the best tasting smoothies.
- Always wash fruits and vegetables thoroughly if using skins.
- Peel fruits and vegetables where necessary, but use skins for additional nutrition such as with apples and carrots.
- Chop ingredients into bite sized pieces suitable to fit your blender or processor.
- Add liquid and softer ingredients first to assist in easy blending.
- Add ice if desired and serve chilled.
- Look for unsweetened milks and juices.
- Although not a good long term solution, use Stevia or similar if desired.

Everyone has different dietary requirements. You may be interested in making your own smoothies as a way to lose weight, manage diabetes, eat low GI foods, have allergies or just want to eat healthy and do a meal replacement when busy. Due to a variety of reasons, the recipes can be modified to suit your own specific needs. You may use a few basic ingredients such as apple, celery and spinach, or a combination of many!

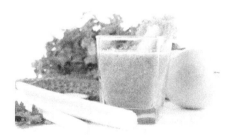

Modify, remove or add ingredients where it makes sense for your own needs.

Milk varieties are wide and varied. Read labels and compare milk types with how much sugar they contain. Some recipes call for almond milk or coconut milk instead of cow's milk. The type of milk is a personal choice and can be interchanged, so experiment. Smoothies are great for weight loss being full of fibre, vitamins and minerals.

If the fruit is too sweet, reduce the quantity you put in, use an alternative fruit, or place more greens or oats into the smoothie. Oatmeal is also a good thickener with only 0.3g of sugar per 100g. **Banana has about 12g of sugar per 100g, apple about 10g and carrot just under 5g.** So carrot may be a good low sugar option as a banana replacement. Remember eating natural fruits in moderation that are freshly prepared by you is good for your health. Get creative, try new things and make the recipe your own!
Another suggestion is to **incorporate super-foods** from time to time into your smoothies to boost your health and well being. Chia seeds, wheatgrass, spinach, oats, Spirulina, flaxseed oil, nuts and wheatgerm are just a few popular additions.

Last thing, where ever possible buy organic and locally.

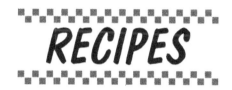

Green Smoothie Blends

Basic Green Smoothie Blend

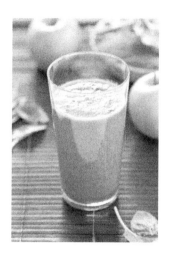

Ingredients:

1 banana

1/2 apple

1 - 2 cups baby spinach leaves

1 cup water or unsweetened coconut water

Directions:

Blend all ingredients for about 10-20 seconds at a time until the desired texture is achieved. Serve chilled. May add a couple of ice cubes when blending.

Green Blackberry Smoothie

Ingredients:

4 cups of baby spinach

2 cups of blackberries

2 cups milk of your choice

3 Tbsp chia seeds

Directions:

This smoothie has fresh and nutty flavor, and the preparation is super-easy. Just blend all ingredients for about 10-20 seconds at a time until the desired texture is achieved. Serve chilled (or just add a couple of ice cubes when blending) and enjoy!

Mango & Kale Green Smoothie

Ingredients:

4 cups of kale leaves

2 cups of large mango chunks

2 cups of ice cold water

1-2 walnuts

Directions:

Mango and kale is an unusual combination that goes together surprisingly well. Blending may take a bit longer than usual, if you choose to add a walnut or two. The choice is yours, but the walnut simply compliments the taste. Just blend everything together and see for yourself. Who knows, maybe this is your next favorite smoothie.

Peggy Annear 2015

Berry Delight

Ingredients:

1 cup unsweetened pomegranate juice

2 cups frozen strawberries

1 cup frozen raspberries

1 cup fresh blueberries or blackberries

1 cup baby spinach leaves

3 Tbsp vanilla flavor protein powder

Directions:

All berries in this recipe, as well as baby spinach leaves and pomegranate juice, have antioxidant properties. Just add some protein powder for energy and vanilla flavor to create this low fat and low carb treat! Always serve your smoothies cold. If you want to drink your smoothie immediately, just add few ice cubes, while blending.

Healing Smoothie

This one packs a punch and isn't for the faint hearted!

Ingredients:

1 cup arugula

1/2 cup pine nuts, soaked

1 carrot, peeled and cut in big chunks

1 sweet pepper, cut in big chunks

1/2 avocado, peeled and pitted

1/2 tomato, cut in big chunks

juice of ½ grapefruit

1 garlic clove

Directions:

Pulse all ingredients in your blender until smooth. Chill before serving. Enjoy this vegetable mix!

Slimming Smoothie

Wheatgrass is high in antioxidants and nutrients.

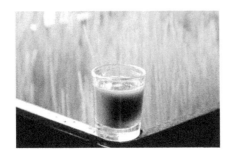

Ingredients:

1 cup spinach leaves or wheatgrass

3 celery stalks

2 apples, cored

1 cucumber

juice of ½ lemon

1 bunch parsley

1 tsp ginger, grated

Directions:

Combine all ingredients in the blender and blend until smooth. This one is a wonderful meal replacement.

Kale Mojito

Ingredients:

2 cups pineapple

2 cups kale (tough stems removed if desired)

2 cups unsweetened coconut water

¼ cup fresh mint leaves

juice of 1 lime

Directions:

How is this for a strange combination? Kale mojito is unusual and very healthy approach to the traditional virgin mojito recipes. Preparing this smoothie is as easy as any other smoothie. Just blend coconut water and kale until smooth. Add remaining ingredients and blend again until smooth. Serve chilled or add some ice at the last phase of blending, or simply use frozen fruit. Enjoy!

Pink Cabbage Glow

Ingredients:

1 cup milk

1 cup cabbage

1 cup strawberries

¼ cup raspberries

1 banana, frozen

1 Tbsp flax seed oil

Directions:

Cabbage? And pink? Yes, this is pink cabbage smoothie, and it still falls into green smoothie category. In fact, don't be afraid of fruit and vegetables coloring your "green" smoothie, this is only natural. The "magical" process of turning green cabbage into pink smoothie, is the same as for all smoothies. Just combine all ingredients in a blender and blend until smooth. Serve chilled, or add ice to the recipe, if desired.

A vegetable fruit smoothie detox wonder full of energy and flavor. If you need sweetener, add some dates.

Green Vegetable Bomb

This recipe was adapted from the book by Jane Burton "Paleo Smoothies"

Ingredients:

1 ripe pear - (cored & cut into chunk size pieces)

1-2 cups seedless grapes of your choice

1 cups washed kale leaves, tough stems removed if prefer

1 cup broccoli florets or kale (lightly steamed to reduce hardness)

1 cup coconut cream (or double cream)

1 cup apple juice

juice of half a lime or lemon

Directions:

Blend all ingredients until smooth. Pour the smoothie into glasses.

Peggy Annear 2015

Green Light Smoothie

Ingredients:

2 cups romaine lettuce, chopped

2 cups spinach, chopped

1/2 cup broccoli, lightly steamed and chopped

1/2 cup water

1/2 apple

1/2 banana

2 Tbsp fresh lemon juice

Directions:

Mix together all ingredients in a blender until smooth. Pour the smoothie in glasses. Bottoms up!

V8 Juice

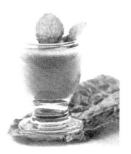

Ingredients:

1¼ cups fresh cubed mango (frozen is okay)

1 cup of chilled orange juice

1¼ cups kale leaf chunks (stems removed)

2 medium sticks of celery

1/4 cup wheatgrass

1/4 cup parsley

1/4cup fresh mint

1/4 cup tomato

1/4 tsp ground or finely grated ginger

1/4 cup red or green capsicum pepper, optional

Directions:

Place liquids into blender, then all other ingredients and blend well.

Refreshing Mango Melon Smoothie

Ingredients:

2 cups unsweetened coconut water

2 cups spinach

1 ½ cups mango, peeled and diced

1 ½ cups watermelon, peeled and diced

Directions:

This smoothie is packed with antioxidants, vitamins A and C and is also delicious. Prepare it by combining all ingredients in blender and blending until smooth. Chill before serving, use frozen fruit or simply add a little bit of ice in the blender while preparing this smoothie. Enjoy!

Cinnaberry Green Smoothie

Ingredients:

2 cups almond milk

2 cups young chard

2 cups frozen berries of your choice

1 banana

¼ tsp ground cinnamon

Directions:

This smoothie combines many classy smoothie ingredients with a dash of cinnamon added for lovely spiciness. Chard should best be used young, as mature leaves tend to get quite bitter and are better used cooked in stews, soups and many other dishes. As for the smoothie, it is prepared by combing all the ingredients in a blender and blended until smooth. If you are using fresh berries, use a frozen banana or add some ice to the recipe, since smoothies taste much better, when served cool.

Peanut Butter and Jelly Smoothie

Ingredients:

2 cups fresh spinach leaves

2 cups almond milk

2 cups seedless red grapes

2 bananas

4 Tbsp unsweetened peanut butter

Directions:

Have you ever craved a peanut butter jelly sandwich, and wondered, if there are any healthier alternatives that would taste the same? Turns out green smoothies can respond even to this craving. This smoothie is more like a meal than a snack, because of the caloric value, but who cares. It makes filling breakfast! Combine all ingredients in a blender, and blend until the texture is thick and smooth. Serve chilled.

Vitamin C Blast

Ingredients:

2 cups kale

1 ½ cup cranberry juice, unsweetened

1 cup shredded ice

2 bananas

2 blood oranges, peeled

1 lime, peeled and seeded

Directions:

Blend cranberry juice, kale, bananas, blood oranges and lime in a blender until smooth. Add ice, cover and blend again until smooth. Serve chilled. Enjoy your boost of vitamin C and antioxidants!

Kiwi Spinach Smoothie

Ingredients:

3 cups baby spinach leaves

1 cup ice cold water or shredded ice

3 kiwis

2 bananas

2 nectarines

Directions:

This smoothie is naturally sweet and healthy. The recipe is simple and perfect for kiwi lovers. Its preparation is the same as for all smoothies. Place all ingredients in a blender. Blend thoroughly, and serve cold!

Vanilla Parsley Smoothie

Ingredients:

1 cup ice cold water or shredded ice

¼ cup parsley, coarsely chopped

¼ cup walnuts

½ avocado

2 Tbsp lime juice

1 vanilla bean or 1 tsp vanilla extract

Directions:

This might seem to be a bit unusual blend of flavors, but surprisingly, it goes well together. If you are using a vanilla bean, cut it in half and with a small knife gently scrape the seeds out of the pod. Place the seeds in a blender. Add water or shredded ice, parsley, walnuts, avocado and lime juice. Blend until smooth. If you want this smoothie to be a bit sweeter, you can add one or two tablespoons honey or similar natural sweetener. Serve cool and enjoy!

Peggy Annear 2015

Green Pumpkin Smoothie

Ingredients:

1 cup spinach leaves

½ cup milk

½ cup plain unsweetened yogurt

½ cup pumpkin puree (from boiled pumpkins)

2 bananas

¼ tsp cinnamon

pinch of allspice

small pinch of ground nutmeg

Directions:

Tastes just like pumpkin pie! It is easy to make your own pumpkin spice from cinnamon, ginger, allspice, cloves, mace and nutmeg. The key spices in the mix are cinnamon, allspice and nutmeg. Just by adding these spices to this pumpkin puree, you'll get the familiar flavor. Making the smoothie itself is even easier. Just puree milk, yogurt and spinach leaves for few seconds in a blender, then add pumpkin puree, bananas and spices.

Coconut Pear Smoothie

Ingredients:

1 cup coconut milk

½ cup shredded ice or ice cubes

½ cup spinach leaves

½ cup kale, roughly chopped

2 pears, peeled, cored and roughly cut

juice of half a lime

Directions:

Combine all ingredients and blend until smooth. If you would like to make your smoothie sweeter, add 1 tablespoon of agave syrup or warmed honey.

Emerald Green Smoothie

Ingredients:

1 cup coconut milk

1 cup kale, stems removed

1 cup baby spinach leaves, washed

½ cup mango, cut into cubes

1 banana, peeled

1/2 tsp chia seeds (optional)

½ cup water

½ cup ice cubes

1 tsp honey or Stevia sweetener optionally.

Directions:

Pour the coconut milk in the blender, then add all the other ingredients. Blend until smooth. Garnish with a baby spinach leaf or halved strawberry for color.

David's Super Smoothie

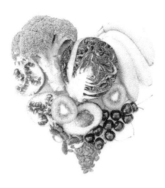

My son's creation before going to work. Be adventurous! Interchange with pomegranate, small amounts of cabbage and broccoli.

Ingredients:

1 cup unsweetened almond milk

1 cup of watermelon or apple

1 banana (cut into pieces)

1 small handful baby spinach leaves or wheatgrass

1 peeled, chopped carrot

1/2 cup water

1 tspn chia seeds (that's almost 2 grams of fibre!)

Directions:

Combine all ingredients in blender and blend on high till smooth. (approx. 2-3 minutes depending on blender) Garnish with a sprig of mint.

Dairy Smoothie Blends

Low GI Oat Drink

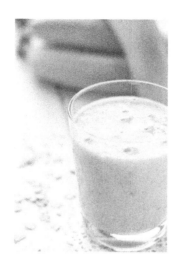

Ingredients:

1/4 cup old-fashioned rolled oats

1/2 cup natural yogurt

1 under ripe banana, cut into thirds

1/2 cup milk or cream

2 tspn honey

1/4 tspn ground cinnamon

Directions:

Combine the oats, yogurt, banana, milk, honey, and cinnamon in your blender. Puree until smooth. You may add ½ cup of orange juice too.

Milky Blackberry Green Smoothie

Ingredients:

4 cups of baby spinach

2 cups of blackberries

2 cups of milk

3 Tbsp chia seeds

Directions:

This smoothie has fresh and nutty flavor, and the preparation is super-easy. Just blend all ingredients for about 10-20 seconds at a time until the desired texture is achieved. Serve chilled (or just add a couple of ice cubes when blending) and enjoy!

Iced Coffee Smoothie

This recipe was inspired by Jane Burton's "Paleo Smoothies" recipe book.

Ingredients:

1 cup good quality brewed coffee, chilled

1/4 cup cream

1/2 tsp vanilla extract

1 heaped Tbsp 100% cacao powder

1 Tbsp raw honey or Stevia (optional sweeteners, mix into the coffee while still warm)

Directions:

Make the coffee, add the honey, then chill. Blend all ingredients together.

Peaches & Cream

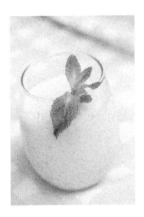

Ingredients:

1 cup milk

½ cup plain non-sweetened yogurt

2 cups fresh peaches or favorite fruit, cut into slices

1 cup crushed ice

Directions:

This recipe actually is 2 in 1. You can blend these ingredients to create a creamy low-fat, low-carb smoothie OR you can use the same ingredients (minus ice) for making smoothie Popsicle. Just pour the mixture in Popsicle moulds or paper cups, add a stick and wait 6 hours or until they're firm. It's up to you to decide, if you'd like to drink your smoothie now or eat it later.

Eggnog Smoothie

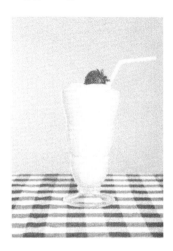

Ingredients:

1 cup coconut cream

1 large egg

1/2 tsp cinnamon

1/2 tsp nutmeg

1/4 tsp vanilla extract

dash of rum (optional)

Directions:

Blend all ingredients. Pour the smoothie into glasses topped with a sprinkle of cinnamon, dob of cream or sliced fruit. Serve chilled and enjoy!

Smoothie Tropicana

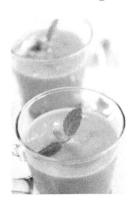

Ingredients:

1 cup milk

½ cup plain low-fat yogurt

1 cup fresh banana, peeled and sliced

1 cup mango, sliced

½ cup shredded ice (or equivalent in ice cubes)

Directions:

In a blender combine milk, yogurt, banana slices and mango slices. Cover and blend until smooth. Add ice, cover and blend until smooth. This smoothie tastes great on a hot, sunny day, when served cold. Just garnish it with mango or lime wedges, close your eyes, and imagine that you are on a tropical island...

Two Color Smoothie

Ingredients:

1 ½ cups watermelon, peel removed, seeded and cut into large chunks

1 cup cantaloupe, peeled and cut into large chunks

½ cup plain, natural low-sugar yogurt

¼ cup orange juice

Directions:

Place watermelon in a blender, cover and blend until smooth. Divide the watermelon puree between two large glasses, and set aside. Clean your blender. Place cantaloupe, yogurt and orange juice in it. Cover and blend until smooth. Now is the tricky part. The second mixture is lighter than the first, but, if you put force when pouring, both parts will mix. In order for your smoothie to be in two colored sections, pour the yogurt/cantaloupe/orange juice mixture slowly and gently into the serving glasses on top of the watermelon puree. If desired, garnish with small cantaloupe wedges.

Almond Cacao Crunch

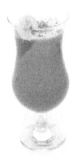

Cacao nibs are highly nutritious and add crunch!

Ingredients:

1/4 cup milk

1/4 cup almonds

1 banana

3 egg whites

1 Tbsp dried carob powder or 100% pure cacao powder

1 tsp cacao nibs (optional)

*Add Stevia or some honey if desired.

Directions:

Combine all ingredients in your blender and pulse until smooth. Serve immediately with a slice of banana and enjoy!

Berry Cocoa Smoothie

Ingredients:

1 cup milk

½ cup blueberries

1 banana, peeled and cut into large chunks

5 large strawberries

1 Tbsp unsweetened cacao powder

2 Tbsp chia seeds, soaked in water (for about 5 minutes)

Directions:

Combine all ingredients in a blender and pulse on high for 20-30 seconds or until you have reached the desired consistency. Serve chilled in a large glass or add a little bit of ice, when blending, if you wish to drink this berrylicious cocoa drink immediately. This smoothie is a great source of vitamins C and A, and it also contains calcium and iron. So much goodness in just one glass!

Sunset Cabbage Blend

Ingredients:

1 cup milk

1 cup cabbage

1 cup strawberries

¼ cup raspberries

1 banana, frozen

1 Tbsp flax seed oil

Directions:

Cabbage? And pink? Yes, this is pink cabbage smoothie, and it still falls into green smoothie category. In fact, don't be afraid of fruit and vegetables coloring your "green" smoothie, this is only natural. The "magical" process of turning green cabbage into pink smoothie, is the same as for all smoothies. Just combine all ingredients in a blender and blend until smooth. Serve chilled, or add ice to the recipe, if desired. Enjoy!

Strawberry Cream Protein Smoothie

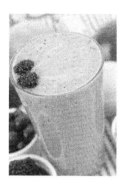

Ingredients:

1 12oz (340g) package soft silken tofu

1 - 2 cups orange juice, chilled

1/2 cup coconut cream or double cream

2/3 - 1 cup strawberries

1 tsp vanilla

Directions:

Tofu is a great protein source, and it is very filling. If you need a smoothie for energy, silken tofu is the way to go! Make sure that the tofu you are purchasing is silken, not regular. If you can't find soft silken tofu, don't worry too much, because firm silken tofu is only slightly firmer than soft. To prepare the smoothie, just combine all ingredients in a blender. As always, serve cold and enjoy!

Green Pumpkin Smoothie

Ingredients:

1 cup spinach leaves

½ cup milk

½ cup plain natural low sugar yogurt

½ cup pumpkin puree (from boiled pumpkins)

2 bananas

¼ tsp cinnamon

pinch of allspice

small pinch of ground nutmeg

Directions:

Tastes just like pumpkin pie! It is easy to make your own pumpkin spice from cinnamon, ginger, allspice, cloves, mace and nutmeg. The key spices in the mix are cinnamon, allspice and nutmeg. Just by adding these spices to this pumpkin puree, you'll get the familiar flavor. Making the smoothie itself is even easier. Just puree milk, yogurt and spinach leaves for few seconds in a blender, then add pumpkin puree, bananas and spices.

Fruit, Vegetable & Protein Smoothie Blends

Carrot and Orange Smoothie

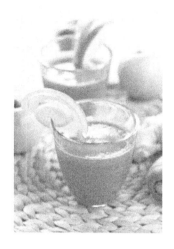

Ingredients:

1 cup orange juice

1 cup carrots, peeled and sliced

1 cup shredded ice

½ tsp orange peel, finely shredded

ginger zest optional

Directions:

In a small saucepan pour a small amount of water, bring it to boil, then add carrot slices. Cook them in boiling water for about 5-10 minutes or until quite tender. Drain well and let them cool. When the carrots have cooled, place them in a blender. Add orange juice and shredded orange peel. Blend until smooth. Add ice cubes, cover your blender and blend until smooth. Serve cold. If you desire, you can use curled orange peels for garnish.

Protein Shake

Ingredients:

1 cup almond milk

3 raw eggs

2 Tbsp water

2 Tbsp honey

juice of ½ lemon

Directions:

Process all ingredients in your blender until smooth.

Sparkling Peach Wine

Ingredients:

1 ½ cups carbonated water, chilled

1 ½ cups shredded ice

3/4 cup coconut water, chilled

3 medium peaches, peeled, pitted and sliced

1 – 2 Tbsp lime juice or lemon juice

Directions:

In a blender combine coconut water, peaches and lime or lemon juice. Cover and blend until smooth. Add ice. Cover and blend until smooth. Spoon the mixture into tall glasses and top with carbonated water. This combines the best properties of smoothies (fruity taste and healthiness and the best properties of lemonade (bubbles, of course).

Carrot Cake Frappe

Ingredients:

1 chilled or frozen banana

1 cup chopped carrots

1 cup coconut cream

1/4 cup crushed walnuts

1/3 cup unsweetened almond milk

1/2 tsp vanilla extract

1 tsp cinnamon

*1 egg (optional)

Directions:

Blend the first 4 ingredients all up together first, mixing well. Then add the remaining ingredients. Add more milk if you prefer. Serve well chilled.

Blueberry Smoothie

Ingredients:

4 cups orange juice

2 cups blueberries or blackberries

1 cup watermelon

Directions:

This recipe can also be used to create low fat/low sugar popsicles. To make a smoothie combine all ingredients in a blender and pulse until smooth. Serve chilled. If you wish to drink this smoothie immediately, add ½ - 1 cup of ice to the recipe. To make smoothie popsicles, pour 2 cups of orange juice evenly in popsicle molds or paper cups. Use the remaining ingredients to create a smoothie. Pour the smoothie slowly in the molds or paper cups. If this is done gently, the purple color will form lovely swirling patterns in the orange juice. Alternatively, you can just simply blend everything together and pour in molds or paper cups. Just put popsicle sticks into each mold or paper cup and freeze for 6 hours or until frozen.

Green Avocado Blaster

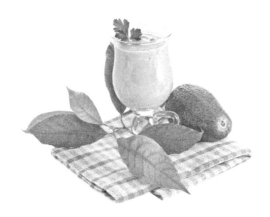

Ingredients:

1 small bunch of spinach

1 tspn cinnamon

1/2 avocado

1/3 banana, frozen

2 ice cubes

1 cup milk

1 scoop Vanilla Shake Powder or Vanilla Essence

Directions:

Put all ingredients into a blender and blend until smooth.

Protein Hot Chocolate

Ingredients:

1 1/2 cups milk, heated

1 egg

1 Tbsp natural, unsweetened peanut butter (or store bought)

2 Tbsp unsweetened cocoa powder

1/2 tsp vanilla extract

1 Tbsp raw honey or Stevia sweetener, heated

(1 Tbsp unsweetened protein powder optional)

Directions:

Heat the milk in a small saucepan over medium heat to a low simmer. Meanwhile combine the egg, peanut butter, protein powder if using, cocoa, vanilla, and warmed honey in blender and mix for 1/2 minute. Gently pour in the hot milk and mix again until smooth, foamy and thick. Serve immediately.

Bloody Mary Smoothie

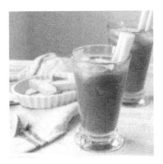

This one takes a little trial and error, some like it, some hate it. Get creative.

Ingredients:

5 ripe tasty tomatoes

1/4 cup seeded cucumber

1 stick of celery, diced

2 - 3 large dates

1 tsp natural Worcestershire sauce

1 apple

juice of one lemon

1 tsp natural horseradish (optional)

1 tsp soy sauce

1 Tbsp vodka

Directions:

Put all ingredients into a blender and blend until smooth.

Spirulina Vanilla Protein Smoothie

Ingredients:

1 cup vanilla soy milk or almond milk

1 tsp Spirulina

1 cup papaya

1 kiwi fruit

1 tsp honey

1/2 tsp cinnamon

Directions:

Blend all together until smooth. Serve chilled.

Strawberry Thick Shake

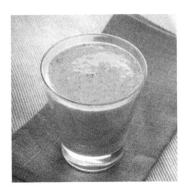

Ingredients:

8 strawberries

1 cup coconut cream

1 - 2 Tbsp honey

2 Tsp vanilla extract

6 cubes ice (crushed)

Directions:

Combine strawberries, cream, honey, vanilla and the ice last. Blend until smooth, thick and creamy. Serve with a sliced strawberry.

Green Tea Smoothie

Ingredients:

3/4 cup strong brewed green tea

1/4 cup almond milk

1 frozen banana

1/2 honeydew melon cut into big chunks

Stevia or 1 tsp honey

Directions:

Blend all ingredients until smooth. Pour the smoothie into glasses.

Super Smoothie

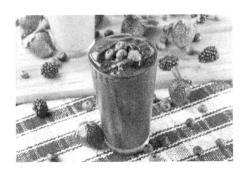

Ingredients:

2 cups frozen berries of your choice

1 cup coconut milk or cream

2/3 cup shredded coconut

1-2 eggs

1/2 Tbsp Chia seeds

Directions:

Place the berries in your blender and pulse them with a dash of hot water to break them easily. Add the coconut shreds, eggs, chia seeds and coconut milk. Blend until smooth. Divide the smoothie into two glasses Bottoms up!

Easy Tomato Squash

Ingredients:

2 tomatoes

3 celery ribs

1 carrot

2 Tbsp fresh lemon juice

Directions:

Combine all ingredients in a blender. Pulse until smooth. If you wish you can add a dash of hot sauce or black pepper to make this smoothie spicier. Bottoms up!

High Protein Smoothie

Ingredients:

1 cup frozen strawberries or blueberries

1 scoop unsweetened protein powder

1 ½ tspn Spirulina powder

1 banana

3 ice cubes

Directions:

Blend all together until smooth. Serve chilled.

Smooth Ruby

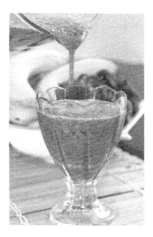

Berries are amongst some of the lowest sugar fruits.

Ingredients:

1½ cups boysenberries and/or raspberries

1 cup strawberries

1 cup blueberries (fresh or frozen)

6 ice crushed ice cubes

squeeze of lemon juice

Directions:

Place all ingredients into blender and process until smooth. Very flexible with amounts. Serve in a parfait glass for that touch of luxury!

Mint Protein Thick Shake

Can substitute water for about 6 ice cubes and banana won't need to be frozen.

Ingredients:

2 cups frozen strawberries or about 15 whole strawberries

1 frozen banana, broken up in chunks

3/4 cup water

3/4 cup unsweetened milk

1/2 cup rolled oats

small handful fresh mint leaves

Directions:

Blend all together until thick and creamy. Serve chilled.

Homemade Coconut Milk Recipe

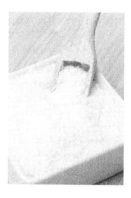

Ingredients:

4 cups of water
2 cups of unsweetened shredded coconut

Directions:

On the stove top, heat the water in a saucepan. You want it hot, but not boiling. Place the coconut into a food processor or blender. If you have a small machine, do this in two batches. Blend for 2 minutes till it has a thick and creamy texture. Now we have to sieve it to get the milk out. Pour the mixture through a mesh colander first to remove most of the coconut. Squeeze what is left through a thin tea-towel or several thicknesses of cheesecloth. This will remove the remaining finer bits of coconut. This may have to be done in batches. If you have to split the water, put all the coconut that you strained out back in the blender, add the remaining water, and repeat. Drink or store in fridge. Home made coconut milk will separate with the thicker bits going to the top, but just shake before using. You can add flavorings too!

Helpful Resources

Juicer Recipes to Treat Common Health Ailments by Jane Burton

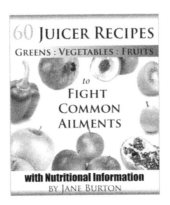

No Sugar Diet & 7 Day Detox Plan by Peggy Annear

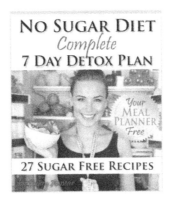

52 Sugar Free Recipes & Sugar Smart Guide by Peggy Annear

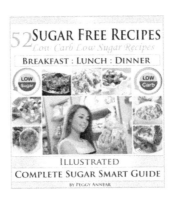

Reviews are important to every author, so if you have enjoyed this book and can spare a minute to leave a review, that would be much appreciated. Thank you.

The End

Notes

Copyright

Made in the USA
Coppell, TX
04 May 2022

77446734R10049